Diabetes and Diet

Diabetes and Diet

The Road to Blood Sugar Control

Jessie White

Dedication

This book is really dedicated to God for His grace and wisdom, my cherished family, the beautiful readers who will find connection inside these pages, and every amazing supporter who paved the way for me. You have led me to this point through your unwavering faith. All readers, especially diabetics, receive a renewal. This book is your travel buddy and your journey is important.

Table of Contents

Acknowledgement

I want to express my heartfelt thanks to God for guiding me throughout the creation of this book. My family's unwavering support and the invaluable contributions of my editor, publisher, and collaborators have shaped its success. To my friends, your constant encouragement has meant the world.

For the amazing picture, a special thanks to vecteezy.com and signos.com.

Furthermore, I want to thank everyone who has read my work and appreciates it very much. I'm glad I got to experience it with you because it's been an amazing ride.

Introduction

"Welcome to 'Diabetes and Diet: The Road to Blood Sugar Control,' a comprehensive guide designed to illuminate the path towards managing diabetes through the remarkable power of your daily food choices.

In a world where health challenges loom large, diabetes stands as an ever-increasing concern. Its reach is profound, affecting millions worldwide. According to the International Diabetes Federation, approximately 463 million people(9.3%) had diabetes in 2019, by 2030 it's expected to increase to 10.2% (578 million) and by 2045, this number is expected to rise to 10.9% (700 million individuals). These statistics paint a stark picture of a global health crisis, demanding a deeper understanding of how to navigate its complexities.

Amidst this health landscape, the role of diet emerges as a beacon of hope, offering a tangible means to not only confront but conquer this formidable condition. Diet plays a pivotal role in the management of diabetes, and this book is your guide to harnessing its power.

This book embarks on a transformative journey, one that unravels the intricate relationship between what you eat and the management of diabetes. It is a journey marked by empowerment, where you are the driver and your plate is your compass. Here, you will embark on a voyage of knowledge, guided by the latest insights from the world of medical science and the wisdom of nutrition.

As we travel this road together, you will discover that managing diabetes through diet is not a mere prescription; it's a celebration of life's flavors, textures, and possibilities. You'll come to understand that your kitchen is a realm of healing, and every meal is a chance to nurture your body and control your blood sugar.

This book is not just about lists of dos and don'ts; it's a narrative of transformation. Each chapter is a stepping stone, offering you the tools, strategies, and understanding needed to craft a diet that aligns with your health goals. From deciphering the intricacies of carbohydrates to exploring the myriad options for tasty, diabetes-friendly recipes, we will cover it all.

By the end of this journey, you will be equipped with knowledge and practical wisdom that empowers you to make informed decisions about what you eat, how you eat, and how to manage your blood sugar levels effectively. 'Diabetes and Diet: The Road to Blood Sugar Control' is more than a book; it's your trusted companion on the path to a healthier, more vibrant life.

So, fasten your seatbelts, for we are about to embark on a voyage where food becomes medicine, choices become empowerment, and diabetes is not an obstacle but a challenge we can overcome. Let's set forth on this road to blood sugar control, and may it be a journey filled with newfound vitality and well-being."

Chapter 1

Understanding Diabetes

What is Diabetes?

According to the WHO, diabetes is a chronic metabolic disorder marked by high blood glucose (also known as blood sugar), which over time causes major harm to the heart, blood vessels, eyes, kidneys, and nerves. The International Diabetes Federation (IDF) describes diabetes as a chronic disease that develops when the body either can't efficiently utilize insulin or the pancreas can no longer produce it.

The hormone insulin, which is produced by the pancreas, functions as a key to allow glucose from food to enter the body's cells where it may be used to make energy. All carbohydrates are converted by the body to glucose in the blood, and insulin aids in the transport of glucose into the cells.

When the body is unable to adequately make or utilize insulin, a condition often known as high blood sugar (hyperglycemia) occurs. Long-term elevated glucose levels are linked to tissue and organ failure, as well as physical harm to the body.

According to the IDF Diabetes Atlas (2021), 10.5% of adults (20–79 years old) have diabetes, with nearly half having no idea that they have the disease.

By 2030, there will be 643 million people living with diabetes, and by 2045, there will be 783 million (an increase of 46%) and 3 out of 4 adults with diabetes reside in low- and middle-income nations.

Types of Diabetes

Diabetes is a complex disease with numerous manifestations. There are a number of additional varieties of diabetes besides the more prevalent ones, such as type 1, type 2, and gestational diabetes, which are as significant.

The three main types of diabetes are:

- Type 1 Diabetes

In type 1 diabetes, the immune system wrongly targets and kills the pancreatic beta cells that produce insulin. Because of this, the hormone needed to control blood sugar (glucose) levels, insulin, is deficient. To control their blood sugar levels and avoid complications, people with Type 1 diabetes need lifelong insulin therapy. It often appears throughout childhood or adolescence, and its precise cause is still not entirely understood.

- Type 2 Diabetes

Type 2 diabetes is a metabolic illness defined by insulin resistance, in which the body's cells do not respond well to insulin and gradually decrease insulin production. High blood sugar levels result from this. Unlike type 1 diabetes, type 2 diabetes is frequently linked to lifestyle factors such as obesity, inactivity, and a poor diet. Though it often appears in adults, younger people are also starting to experience it more frequently. Altering one's lifestyle, taking oral medications, and occasionally using insulin therapy are all possible forms of treatment.

- Gestational Diabetes

Gestational diabetes is a form of diabetes that appears during pregnancy. It happens when the body is unable to manufacture enough insulin to meet the higher demands brought on by the hormonal changes associated with pregnancy. High blood sugar levels result from this. Gestational diabetes can increase the risk of difficulties for the mother and the fetus during pregnancy, although it typically goes away after childbirth. Dietary adjustments, blood sugar monitoring, and occasionally medication or insulin therapy under physician supervision are all normal components of managing gestational diabetes.

Others include:

- Maturity Onset Diabetes of the Young (MODY)

The term mature onset diabetes of the young (MODY) describes a collection of uncommon hereditary types of diabetes that are frequently inherited in an autosomal dominant manner. Unlike the more prevalent kinds of diabetes, MODY often manifests before the age of 25 and is brought on by mutations in particular genes that impact insulin secretion and synthesis. It's possible that people with MODY can occasionally control their illness without insulin therapy by changing their diet or lifestyle. Depending on whatever genetic MODY subtype a person has, different treatment approaches may be used.

- Latent Autoimmune Diabetes in Adults (LADA)

LADA, commonly known as "type 1.5 diabetes," is a kind of diabetes that has characteristics of both type 1 and type 2 diabetes.. LADA often manifests in adulthood and initially has moderate symptoms and a slow start with type 2 diabetes. Similar to type 1 diabetes, it is brought on by an autoimmune reaction that gradually destroys the pancreatic beta cells that produce insulin.

As their insulin production declines over time, persons with LADA typically need insulin therapy to control their blood sugar levels. Due to its adult onset and moderate presenting features, LADA is initially frequently misdiagnosed as Type 2 diabetes, but its autoimmune nature distinguishes it. To provide proper treatment for LADA, a correct diagnosis is essential.

- Neonatal Diabetes

It is an unusual kind of diabetes that develops within the first six months of life. Genetic changes that impact the pancreas' growth and operation, particularly the insulin-producing beta cells, are the root cause.

There are two types of neonatal diabetes:
- Transient, and
- Permanent.

Within the first few months of life, transient neonatal diabetes often improves or disappears, and those who are affected may not require lifetime therapy. On the other hand, permanent neonatal diabetes necessitates lifelong administration of insulin therapy. Genetic testing is frequently used to pinpoint the precise genetic mutation responsible for the ailment, which can assist doctors choose the best course of action.

- Wolfram Syndrome

Wolfram Syndrome is a rare hereditary condition also referred to as DIDMOAD (Diabetes Insipidus, Diabetes Mellitus, Optic Atrophy, and Deafness). It predominantly affects the nervous system and can cause hearing loss, diabetes mellitus, diabetes insipidus, and a variety of neurological symptoms. It can also cause problems with eyesight owing to optic atrophy. Mutations in the WFS1 or CISD2 genes are the root cause. Since this illness has no known treatment, management usually entails focusing on the individual symptoms and offering supportive care. Effective management of the illness depends on an early diagnosis and a multidisciplinary approach to care.

- Alström Syndrome

Alström Syndrome is an extremely rare genetic disorder that affects multiple organ systems in the body. It is caused by mutations in the ALMS1 gene. Individuals with Alström Syndrome often experience a range of symptoms including vision and hearing problems, obesity, insulin resistance leading to diabetes, heart and liver issues, and hormonal imbalances. This syndrome can vary widely in its presentation and severity. Management involves addressing the various medical issues as they arise and providing supportive care. Due to its complexity, a multidisciplinary medical approach is typically required to manage the condition effectively.

- Type 3c diabetes

Type 3c diabetes, commonly referred to as pancreatogenic diabetes or secondary diabetes, is a type of diabetes brought on by pancreatic injury or disease. This can include illnesses including cystic fibrosis, chronic pancreatitis, pancreatic cancer, and other pancreatic abnormalities. Diabetes develops as a result of the pancreas' diminished capacity to make insulin. Unlike type 1 and type 2 diabetes, type 3c diabetes is caused by pancreatic dysfunction rather than autoimmune conditions or insulin resistance. The standard course of management includes treating the underlying pancreatic disorder in addition to treating the diabetes with the proper medicines or insulin therapy.

- Steroid-induced diabetes

Steroid-induced diabetes, sometimes referred to as corticosteroid-induced diabetes or steroid diabetes, is a kind of diabetes that appears after long-term or high-dose corticosteroid treatment. These drugs are frequently used to treat autoimmune diseases, various inflammatory illnesses, and specific cancers. Because steroids decrease the body's sensitivity to insulin and cause the liver to produce more glucose, they can cause blood sugar levels to rise.

The chance of acquiring steroid-induced diabetes may be higher in people who are already at risk for the disease. Monitoring blood sugar levels carefully, changing the steroid dosage when necessary, and, occasionally, using insulin or diabetes drugs to manage blood sugar levels while receiving steroid treatment are all part of management. Some people may see a return to normal blood sugar levels once steroid use is stopped or reduced.

- Cystic fibrosis diabetes

Cystic fibrosis-related diabetes (CFRD) is a special kind of diabetes that only affects people with cystic fibrosis (CF), a hereditary disease that predominantly affects the digestive and respiratory systems. Inflammatory fibrosis of the pancreas (CFRD) is brought on by the accumulation of thick, gummy mucus, which can harm insulin-producing cells and decrease insulin release. Diabetes is therefore more likely to occur in CF patients.

Type 1 and type 2 diabetes share similarities with CFRD. Depending on the demands of the individual, it might need to be managed with insulin, but the specifics can change. To assist control CF and overall health, it is essential to regularly monitor blood sugar levels. Treatment also entails keeping blood sugar levels steady. Specialists in CF and diabetes are frequently included on Cystic Fibrosis Care Teams to offer complete care and support to CFRD patients.

Signs and Symptoms

The signs and symptoms of diabetes can vary depending on the type of diabetes and its severity.

Here are common signs and symptoms:

1. *Frequent Urination*: You may find yourself urinating more often than usual, particularly at night (nocturia).

2. *Excessive Thirst*: Increased urination can lead to excessive thirst as your body tries to compensate for fluid loss.

3. *Unexplained Weight Loss*: Despite eating normally or even more, unexplained weight loss can occur, especially in type 1 diabetes.

4. *Increased Hunger*: You might feel hungry more frequently, especially if your body is not effectively using glucose for energy.

5. *Fatigue*: Diabetes can lead to fatigue and a general sense of weakness due to inefficient glucose utilization.

6. *Blurred Vision*: High blood sugar levels can cause changes in the shape of the eye's lens, leading to blurred vision.

7. *Slow Healing*: Wounds, cuts, or sores may take longer to heal in individuals with diabetes.

8. *Tingling or Numbness*: Nerve damage (neuropathy) can cause tingling, numbness, or pain in the hands and feet.

9. *Recurrent Infections*: High blood sugar can weaken the immune system, making you more susceptible to infections, especially in areas like the urinary tract, skin, or gums.

10. *Itchy Skin*: Dry or itchy skin, particularly around the genitals, can be a symptom.

11. *Gum Problems*: Diabetes can increase the risk of gum disease.

12. *Yeast Infections*: Women with diabetes might experience more frequent yeast infections.

Type 1 Diabetes

Typically, the symptoms of type 1 diabetes develop rapidly, often over a few weeks. This type is more common in children and young adults.

Type 2 Diabetes

The symptoms of type 2 diabetes may develop more gradually and may not be as noticeable. Many people with type 2 diabetes have no symptoms initially.

If you experience any of these symptoms, especially if they persist or worsen, it's important to see a healthcare professional for evaluation and appropriate testing. Early diagnosis and management are essential to prevent complications associated with diabetes.

Diagnosis

In order to identify if someone has diabetes, classify the condition's kind, and gauge its severity, several tests and evaluations are used to diagnose the disease.

Here's an overview of the diagnostic process:

1. *Fasting Blood Sugar Test* (FBS): A fasting blood sugar test measures blood glucose levels after an overnight fast. A fasting blood sugar level of 126 milligrams per deciliter (mg/dL) or higher on two separate occasions typically indicates diabetes.

2. *Oral Glucose Tolerance Test* (OGTT): This test involves fasting overnight and then drinking a sugary solution. Blood sugar levels are checked at intervals over the next few hours. A blood sugar level of 200 mg/dL or higher two hours after the drink suggests diabetes.

3. *A1C Test*: The A1C test provides an average of blood sugar levels over the past two to three months. An A1C level of 6.5% or higher is often used for a diabetes diagnosis.

4. *Random Blood Sugar Test*: If you have symptoms of diabetes (e.g., extreme thirst, frequent urination), a random blood sugar test can be done at any time of the day without fasting. A blood sugar level of 200 mg/dL or higher along with diabetes symptoms may indicate diabetes.

5. *Glycated Albumin* (GA) *Test*: This test measures blood sugar control over the past few weeks and can be useful in certain situations.

6. *C-Peptide Test*: This test measures the level of C-peptide in the blood, which can help differentiate between type 1 and type 2 diabetes. Low C-peptide levels may suggest type 1 diabetes.

7. *Autoantibody Tests*: These tests can be used to detect antibodies associated with autoimmune type 1 diabetes.

8. *Physical Examination*: Your healthcare provider may perform a physical examination to look for signs of diabetes-related complications and assess overall health.

9. *Medical History*: Providing a detailed medical history, including family history of diabetes and any symptoms you've been experiencing, is important for diagnosis.

10. *Additional Tests*: Depending on the situation, your healthcare provider may order other tests to evaluate your overall health and any potential complications associated with diabetes, such as kidney function tests, lipid profile, and eye examinations.

It's important to note that a diabetes diagnosis is based on a combination of these tests and clinical evaluation. If you receive a diabetes diagnosis, your healthcare provider will work with you to develop a personalized treatment plan and provide guidance on managing the condition. Regular monitoring and follow-up appointments are essential for ongoing diabetes management.

Chapter 2

Management of Diabetes

Diabetes is a significant medical illness that, over time, can make you feel extremely hungry and exhausted, among other troubling symptoms. If you do not control this condition, you may experience more significant side effects, including visual loss, dementia, and renal difficulties.

The term "management of diabetes" refers to a comprehensive plan and set of techniques used to keep healthy blood sugar levels in diabetics. It involves doing various things to prevent issues, improve your overall health, and make sure your blood sugar stays where it should be.

Below are the ways to manage this condition

1. Monitor Blood Sugar Levels

Regularly check your blood sugar levels as advised by your healthcare provider. Monitoring helps you understand how your actions affect your blood sugar and allows for timely adjustments to your treatment plan.

2. Healthy Eating

Follow a balanced diet that includes a variety of foods like fruits, vegetables, whole grains, lean proteins, and healthy fats.

- Monitor carbohydrate intake and distribute it evenly throughout the day.
- Consider portion control to manage calorie intake and blood sugar levels.

3. Regular Physical Activity

- Engage in regular exercise, as it can help lower blood sugar, improve insulin sensitivity, and support weight management.
- Aim for at least 150 minutes of moderate-intensity aerobic activity per week, along with strength training exercises.

4. Medications and Insulin Therapy

- Take prescribed medications, including insulin, if recommended by your healthcare provider.
- Ensure proper dosing and timing of medications or insulin injections.

5. Stress Management

- Practice stress-reduction techniques such as mindfulness, meditation, yoga, or deep breathing exercises.
- High stress levels can impact blood sugar levels.

6. Regular Healthcare Check-ups

Attend regular appointments with your healthcare team to monitor your overall health, review your diabetes management plan, and make necessary adjustments.

7. Foot Care

- Inspect your feet daily for any cuts, sores, or blisters. Report any issues to your healthcare provider.
- Keep your feet clean and moisturized.

8. Eye and Dental Care

Visit eye and dental specialists regularly for check-ups, as diabetes can increase the risk of eye and dental problems.

9. Weight Management

- If overweight, work with your healthcare team to set realistic weight loss goals and strategies.

Achieving and maintaining a healthy weight can improve blood sugar control.

10. Education and Support

Learn about diabetes management through educational programs, books, or online resources. Join support groups to connect with others who have diabetes and share experiences.

11. Emergency Preparedness

Develop a plan for handling hypoglycemia (low blood sugar) and hyperglycemia (high blood sugar) emergencies.

12. Blood Pressure and Cholesterol Control

Manage blood pressure and cholesterol levels through medications and lifestyle changes to reduce the risk of heart disease, a common complication of diabetes.

13. Vaccinations

Stay up-to-date with vaccinations, including the flu and pneumonia vaccines, to protect against infections that can affect blood sugar control.

14. Medication Adherence

Take your medications as prescribed by your healthcare provider. Consistency is crucial for managing diabetes effectively.

15. Self-Care and Advocacy

Take an active role in your health by advocating for your needs and seeking necessary healthcare services.

Remember that diabetes management is a lifelong journey, and it's important to work closely with your healthcare team to create a personalized plan tailored to your specific needs and circumstances.

The Role of Diet in Diabetes Management

Diet plays a crucial role in managing diabetes by helping to control blood sugar levels and improve overall health.

Here's the role of diet in diabetes management:

1. Carbohydrate Management

Carbohydrates have the most significant impact on blood sugar levels. Managing carbohydrate intake is a fundamental part of diabetes control.

As it:

- Empowers individuals with diabetes to take control of their blood sugar levels
- Reduces the risk of complications, and
- Improves overall well-being.

You have to:

- Monitor and control portion sizes of carbohydrate-rich foods like bread, rice, pasta, and sugary snacks.
- Consider carbohydrate counting to help match your insulin or medication doses with your food intake.

2. Balanced Nutrition

In order to meet the body's nutritional demands for overall health and wellbeing, balanced nutrition involves ingesting a range of foods in the proper quantities. Aim for a balanced diet that includes a variety of foods, such as fruits, vegetables, whole grains, lean proteins, and healthy fats.

Such a diet can help:

- maintain a healthy weight,
- reduce the risk of chronic diseases like heart disease and diabetes,
- support strong bones and muscles, and
- promote cognitive function.

This balanced approach provides essential nutrients (carbohydrates, proteins, fats and oil, vitamins and minerals) while helping to stabilize blood sugar levels.

3. Fiber-Rich Foods

Foods high in dietary fiber, like whole grains, legumes, and vegetables, can help:

- Slow the absorption of glucose and improve blood sugar control
- Improve insulin sensitivity
- Promote satiety and weight management
- Support gut health
- Reduce cardiovascular risk, and providing a steady source of energy

4. Low-Glycemic Index (GI) Foods

Choose foods with a low GI, as they have a slower and more gradual effect on blood sugar levels.

- They help stabilize blood sugar levels
- Provides sustained energy
- Aids in weight management
- Promotes heart health, and
- Improves mood and mental health.

Examples include whole grains, non-starchy vegetables, and most fruits in moderation.

5. Sugar Control

Sugar control is the process of managing and regulating blood sugar (glucose) levels within a healthy range, especially in the setting of diabetes. This is essential for maintaining general health and avoiding problems brought on by high or low blood sugar.

It can help reduce the risk of complications, such as

- cardiovascular disease,
- nerve damage,
- kidney problems, and
- vision issues.

You have to:

- Limit added sugars in your diet, including sugary beverages, sweets, and desserts. Opt for sugar substitutes if necessary.
- Be mindful of hidden sugars in processed foods.

6. Regular Meal Timing

The term "regular meal timing" describes the habit of having meals and snacks at regular intervals throughout the day. It entails creating a schedule so that you eat around the same times every day. As an illustration, eating breakfast, lunch, and dinner at regular intervals with planned snacks in between is an example of regular meal timing.

Regular meal timing plays a pivotal role in diabetes management by:

- stabilizing blood sugar levels,
- facilitating insulin management,
- preventing hypoglycemia,
- improving glycemic control,
- aiding weight management,
- enhancing medication effectiveness,
- allowing for predictable blood sugar responses to food, and
- seamlessly integrating into daily lifestyles.

This practice assists individuals in achieving better blood sugar regulation and reducing the risk of complications associated with diabetes, with personalized guidance from healthcare providers or dietitians being crucial for effective implementation.

7. Portion Control

Portion control refers to managing the size and quantity of food you consume during meals and snacks. It's an essential aspect of maintaining a balanced and healthy diet.

It helps:

- regulate blood sugar levels,
- manage weight, and
- achieve better overall glycemic control.

8. Healthy Fats

Unsaturated fats, commonly referred to as healthy fats, are a type of dietary fat that, when consumed in moderation, have a number of health advantages. They are regarded as "healthy" because they can promote general health and lower the risk of developing specific chronic diseases.

Here are the functions of healthy fats in diabetes management:
- Blood Sugar Regulation
- Improved Insulin Sensitivity
- Heart Health
- Satiety and Weight Management
- Anti-Inflammatory Effects
- Blood Pressure Control
- Reduced Risk of Complications

You have to:

- Include sources of healthy fats, such as avocados, nuts, seeds, and olive oil, in your diet for heart health.
- Limit saturated and Trans fats, which can contribute to heart disease.

9. Protein Moderation

A crucial part of managing diabetes is moderate protein intake. Protein moderation refers to consuming an appropriate amount of protein in your diet, neither too little nor too much, to meet your nutritional needs and health goals.

It does the followings:

- It aids in blood sugar control by preventing rapid glucose spikes after meals,
- while its filling nature supports appetite regulation and weight management, both essential for diabetes care
- Aids in maintaining muscle health, a key player in glucose metabolism.
- It stimulates the release of glucagon, helping prevent hypoglycemia and ensuring steady energy levels between meals.

Therefore you need to:

- Consume lean sources of protein, like poultry, fish, tofu, and legumes.

- Avoid excessive protein intake, as it can be converted into glucose in the body.

10. Hydration

Hydration is the process of giving your body the right amount of fluid, usually in the form of water, to keep it operating as it should. Hydration plays a crucial role in diabetes management namely:

- helps maintain stable blood sugar levels, as dehydration can lead to higher blood sugar concentrations, making it more challenging to manage diabetes
- aids medication efficacy as many diabetes medications work more effectively when you are well-hydrated
- supports kidney function, which is vital for filtering blood and removing waste products
- prevents diabetes-related complications, such as diabetic ketoacidosis (DKA) or hyperosmolar hyperglycemic state (HHS), which are brought about by dehydration
- aids in weight management, which is important for many people with diabetes, as obesity is a risk factor for type 2 diabetes.
- balances electrolytes like sodium and potassium, which is crucial for overall health, especially in people with diabetes.

Note: Diabetes can cause increased thirst (polydipsia), which may lead to more fluid intake. It's important for people with diabetes to monitor their fluid intake to ensure they are drinking enough without overdoing it.

To promote optimal hydration in diabetes control, it's also critical to:

- Drink water consistently throughout the day and pay attention to your body's thirst cues.
- Avoid sugary drinks and excessive caffeine.
- keep an eye on blood sugar levels and alter insulin or medicine dosage as needed, particularly in hot weather or when exercising.

For tailored hydration advice, people with diabetes should speak with a healthcare professional or registered dietitian.

Individualization

Work with a registered dietitian or healthcare provider to create a personalized meal plan that takes into account your specific needs, preferences, and any other medical conditions.

Regular Monitoring

Monitor blood sugar levels before and after meals to understand how different foods affect your body. Adjust your diet as needed.

Education and Support

Learn about nutrition and diabetes management through educational programs or counseling. Join support groups to share experiences and strategies with others managing diabetes.

Diet is a powerful tool for managing diabetes, but it's important to remember that individual responses to foods can vary. Regular communication with your healthcare team and a registered dietitian is essential for creating and maintaining a diabetes-friendly eating plan tailored to your unique needs.

Chapter 3

Blood Sugar and Its Impact

Blood sugar, or glucose, is like the body's energy currency. It's the fuel that keeps your cells, muscles, organs, and brain working smoothly. But, like managing money, your body needs to keep a close eye on blood sugar levels to avoid trouble.

Imagine high blood sugar as overspending. If it stays too high for too long, it can lead to problems like diabetes and heart issues. It's like maxing out your credit card – not good in the long run. On the flip side, low blood sugar is like running out of cash. It can make you feel shaky and dizzy, and if it drops too low, you might even pass out.

That's why your body has special hormones, like insulin and glucagon, to help keep blood sugar in check. Insulin lowers it when it's too high, and glucagon raises it when it's too low.

So, just like managing your finances, keeping an eye on your blood sugar through a healthy diet, exercise, and sometimes medication is essential for a balanced and healthy life.

How Blood Sugar Affects Health

Your general health has a lot to do with your blood sugar levels. Things go easily when they're in the right range. But when they aren't in harmony, it can cause a number of health problems.

Let's take a look:

1. Risk of Diabetes

When you consistently have high levels of sugar in your bloodstream (often due to poor diet and lifestyle habits), your cells may not respond well to insulin anymore. They become somewhat resistant to its effects. This means glucose has a hard time entering your cells, and as a result, your blood sugar levels stay elevated. This consistent high blood sugar levels can increase the risk of developing type 2 diabetes.

2. Heart Health

Prolonged high blood sugar levels,

- can damage the inner lining of blood vessels. This damage makes it easier for fatty deposits, like cholesterol, to accumulate on the vessel walls.
- can (that is the accumulation of fatty deposits) lead to the formation of plaques thereby resulting in atherosclerosis (arteries become narrow and stiffened).

As the plague grows, it can severely restrict the flow of blood via the arteries and this can lead to cardiovascular problems like

- Coronary Artery Disease (CAD): When the arteries that supply blood to the heart muscle become narrowed or blocked by plaques, it can result in chest pain (angina) or even a heart attack.

- Peripheral Artery Disease (PAD): Plaque buildup in the arteries of the arms and legs can lead to pain, numbness, and reduced circulation in these extremities.

- Stroke: If plaques form in the arteries supplying the brain, they can increase the risk of a stroke by disrupting blood flow to parts of the brain.

3. Energy Levels

Balanced blood sugar levels help maintain steady energy throughout the day. When levels are too high or too low, it can result in energy crashes and fatigue. It's important to have a balanced diet and monitor sugar intake to help regulate blood sugar effectively.

4. Weight Management

High blood sugar can have a significant impact on your eating habits and your weight. It can also disrupt hormones that regulate hunger and satiety.

- *Overeating*: It can cause desires for foods high in sugar and calories when your blood sugar levels are persistently high. These foods and desserts may become more appealing to you. Because your body is having trouble utilizing the glucose for energy, this can result in overeating.

- *Weight Gain*: Overeating can result in consuming too many calories, especially those from sugary or high-carb foods, which can eventually lead to weight gain. The body frequently stores these additional calories as fat.

- *Hormonal Disruption*: Hormones that control hunger and satiety can become abnormally active when blood sugar levels are high. As an illustration, it may cause insulin resistance, which is a condition in which your body does not react favorably to insulin. Normal functions of insulin include regulating blood sugar and regulating appetite. You could continue to feel hungry even after eating when it's not functioning properly.

- *Vicious Cycle*: Weight gain can worsen insulin resistance, creating a cycle where high blood sugar levels lead to overeating, which in turn leads to more weight gain and higher blood sugar levels.

5. Nerve Damage

Prolonged high blood sugar can damage nerves, causing numbness, tingling, and pain, particularly in the hands and feet.

6. Kidney Function

Elevated blood sugar can strain the kidneys over time, potentially leading to kidney damage or even failure.

This includes:

- Increased workload, where the kidneys are required to filter more blood to remove the excess glucose, thereby stressing the kidneys.
- damage the small blood vessels within the kidneys. Over time, this can impair their ability to function properly.
- Diabetic nephropathy (a form of kidney disease specific to diabetes). In its early stages, it may not cause noticeable symptoms. However, over time, it can progress to kidney damage or even kidney failure.
- High blood pressure (hypertension), which is another factor that can harm the kidneys.

7. Vision Issues

High blood sugar levels can indeed lead to several vision issues, primarily due to the damage they cause to the blood vessels in the eyes.

Some common vision problems associated with diabetes are:

- Diabetic Retinopathy
- Diabetic Macular Edema (DME)
- Cataracts
- Glaucoma
- Blurred Vision

8. Infection Risk

High blood sugar can weaken the immune system, making it harder for the body to fight infections.

This occurs because elevated blood sugar can

- impair the function of white blood cells, which are crucial for fighting off bacteria and viruses
- slow down wound healing in diabetes and as a result, it creates entry points for pathogens, increasing the risk of infections
- disrupts the balance of gut bacteria, essential for immune function,

As a result, people with diabetes are more vulnerable to infections like

- urinary tract infections,
- skin infections, and
- fungal infections.

Effective blood sugar management, proper hygiene practices, and regular healthcare check-ups are vital to minimize this heightened infection risk.

9. Mood and Mental Health

Diabetes can have a substantial impact on mood and mental health due to fluctuating blood sugar levels. This can result in:

- anger,
- mood swings, and
- difficulties concentrating

Hypoglycemia, or low blood sugar, can make you tense and irritable, while hyperglycemia, or excess blood sugar, can cause

- mood changes and

- even make you feel depressed. It may be difficult to concentrate and make judgments as a result of these variations in mood

- constantly worrying about blood sugar levels can lead to anxiety and stress, and ongoing unpredictability raises the risk of depression. Underscoring the comprehensive approach to diabetes care, sustaining stable mood and mental well-being depends on effective blood sugar management through medication, dietary changes, and lifestyle modifications.

10. Healing Process

High blood sugar can slow down the body's ability to heal wounds, increasing the risk of infections and complications.

11. Long-Term Complications

Uncontrolled high blood sugar over time can lead to serious complications like heart disease, stroke, nerve damage, kidney disease, and vision problems.

On the other hand, low blood sugar can lead to immediate symptoms like shakiness, confusion, and even loss of consciousness. It's important to strike a balance and maintain blood sugar within a healthy range through a combination of proper diet, exercise, medication (if necessary), and regular monitoring. If you have concerns about your blood sugar, consulting a healthcare professional is a smart move.

Target Blood Sugar Ranges

Target blood sugar ranges can vary depending on whether you have diabetes or not. Here are the general target blood sugar ranges for different situations:

For People without Diabetes

- Fasting Blood Sugar (before meals):
  Typically below 100 (70 - 99) mg/dL (3.9 - 5.5 mmol/L).
- Blood Sugar 2 Hours After Eating (postprandial):
  Usually below 140 mg/dL (7.8 mmol/L).

For People with Diabetes

- Fasting Blood Sugar:
  Often between 80 and 130 mg/dL (4.4 - 7.2 mmol/L).
- Blood Sugar Before Meals:
  Typically between 80 and 130 mg/dL.
- Blood Sugar 1-2 Hours After Meals:
  Usually less than 180 mg/dL (10.0 mmol/L).

Fasting blood sugar levels between 100 and 125 mg/dl are a sign of prediabetes, which is a condition where blood sugar levels are higher than "normal" but not yet high enough to be classified as diabetes.

After meal (someone without diabetes)
- 140 mg/dl or less is considered normal blood sugar.
- Prediabetes is between 140 and 199 mg/dl,
- While diabetes is indicated by a blood sugar level of 200 mg/dl or greater.

However, it's important to note that individualized target ranges can vary based on factors like age, overall health, and the type of diabetes (type 1 or type 2). Your healthcare provider will work with you to establish specific target ranges that are right for your situation.

Regular monitoring and working closely with your healthcare team are crucial for managing blood sugar effectively, especially if you have diabetes. They can help you set personalized targets and make necessary adjustments to your treatment plan to keep your blood sugar within a healthy range.

Chapter 4

Managing Blood Sugar Levels

Think of your body as a vehicle that requires gasoline to function properly. Your body's "fuel" is your blood sugar, and just like you wouldn't want to fill the tank too much or too little with gas, you don't want to do either. You feel invigorated and prepared to take on the world when your blood sugar levels are just right. However, it feels as though the car sputters and slows down if they are too high (like pouring too much gas) or too low (like not enough gas).

Therefore, controlling blood sugar is all about maintaining a constant fuel level to prevent unexpected energy dips and fatigue. This entails selecting wholesome meals and snacks and keeping an eye out for sugary items that may disrupt your energy levels.

There are several ways to manage blood sugar levels effectively. They are as follows:

1. Balanced Diet

A balanced diet is unquestionably a key component of optimal health. Your body gets the fundamental building blocks it requires to perform at its best when you include a variety of nutrient-rich foods in your meals. Whole grains, such brown rice and whole wheat, provide long-lasting energy and important fiber that supports digestion. Muscle development and repair are supported by lean proteins like those found in chicken, fish, and lentils. For heart health and proper brain function, it is essential to consume healthy fats, which may be found in foods like avocados, almonds, and olive oil.

Aside from that, the vivid hues of fruits and vegetables signal the presence of numerous vitamins, minerals, and antioxidants that support health and illness prevention. You may protect yourself against the negative consequences of blood sugar spikes, weight gain, and an increased risk of chronic illnesses by avoiding excessive amounts of sugar and refined carbs, which are frequently present in sugary snacks and sugary drinks.

Your dedication to keeping this balance in your food is an investment in your wellbeing, encouraging vigor, toughness, and general lifespan. Never forget that taking tiny efforts toward a better diet can have a big impact over time. It's a path toward nourishing your body and cultivating peace with food.

2. Portion Control

Portion control is important to avoid overeating, which can lead to blood sugar rises. By managing your portions, you can reduce your calorie intake and maintain a healthy weight. Therefore, maintaining a healthy weight helps prevent type 2 diabetes and has been shown to lower blood sugar levels.

For regulating portion amounts, consider the following advice:

- Count and weigh your servings.
- Utilize smaller plates.
- Do not eat at all-you-can-eat establishments (restaurants).
- Examine the portion amounts and food labels.
- Eat slowly and keep a food diary.

3. Frequent Meals

Of course, maintaining stable blood sugar levels can benefit from eating smaller, well-balanced meals at regular intervals throughout the day. This strategy can lessen significant blood sugar swings, which is crucial for people who are managing diseases like diabetes. Your body receives a continuous supply of nutrients and energy by spreading out your meals, which might help you maintain better blood sugar control.

To maintain general health and sustained energy levels, always remember to include a combination of carbohydrates, proteins, and healthy fats in your meals. Always seek the advice of a qualified healthcare provider or certified dietitian for individualized advice based on your unique requirements.

4. Carb Counting

Your blood sugar levels are significantly influenced by the amount of carbohydrates you consume. Carbohydrates are transformed by your body into sugars, primarily glucose. Insulin then facilitates the consumption and storage of the glucose for energy. This process fails and blood sugar levels can increase when you consume too many carbohydrates or when you have issues with insulin function.

Because of this, the American Diabetes Association (ADA) advises patients with diabetes to control their carb consumption by keeping track of their intake and calculating their required intake of carbohydrates. According to certain research, this can assist you in making wise food plans, which will further enhance blood sugar control. Additionally, numerous studies demonstrate how a low-carb diet lowers blood sugar levels and prevents blood sugar rises.

5. Regular Exercise

Your muscles can use blood sugar for energy and contraction when you exercise often. Exercise will help you maintain a healthy weight and improve your insulin sensitivity. As a result of the improved insulin sensitivity, your cells will be better able to utilize the sugar in your bloodstream. In addition, researchers advice taking part in so-called "exercise snacks" to lower blood sugar and avoid the harm that prolonged sitting might cause. It means simply breaking up your sitting time for a few minutes every 30 minutes during the day with exercise snacks is all that is required. Light, brisk walking or easy resistance workouts like squats or leg raises are a few of the exercises advised.

6. Hydration

You may be able to maintain healthy blood sugar levels by drinking enough water. Additionally to avoiding dehydration, it aids in the kidneys' ability to eliminate any extra sugar in the urine. According to a study of observational studies, people who drank more water were less likely to experience high blood sugar levels. Regular water consumption may rehydrate the blood, lower blood sugar levels, and lower the chance of developing diabetes. Remember that the greatest beverages are water and others with no calories. Avoid products that are sugar-sweetened as they can elevate blood sugar, cause weight gain, and raise the chance of developing diabetes.

7. Stress Management

Your blood sugar levels may be impacted by stress. Blood sugar levels rise as a result of your body secreting the chemicals glucagon and cortisol in response to stress. Exercise, relaxation, and meditation were found to dramatically lower stress and blood sugar levels in one study involving a group of students. People with chronic diabetes may also benefit from exercises and relaxation techniques like yoga and mindfulness-based stress reduction.

8. Adequate Sleep

It feels great and is essential for good health to get adequate sleep. In reality, a lack of sleep and poor sleeping patterns can have an impact on insulin sensitivity and blood sugar levels, raising the risk of type 2 diabetes. They may also stimulate hunger and encourage weight gain. In addition, sleep loss increases cortisol levels, which are crucial for controlling blood sugar levels. Both quantity and quality of sleep are important for healthy functioning. Adults should receive at least 7-8 hours of good sleep each night, according to the National Sleep Foundation.

Here are a few things to do in order to have a better night's sleep:
- Maintain a sleep pattern
- Stay away from coffee and alcohol
- Limit your naps in the afternoon
- Engage in regular exercise, and reduce your screen time before night
- Create a nighttime ritual
- Avoid working in your bedroom
- Take a warm bath or shower before going to bed, and try guided imagery or meditation.

9. Medication and Insulin

Regarding medication and insulin, it is crucial that you follow your doctor's advice in order to maintain good health. Maintaining consistency in dosage and time while using these therapies strictly as directed is essential. You may ensure that your condition is well-controlled and lower the likelihood of problems by doing this. Additionally, it is essential to communicate with your doctor frequently; any queries or worries you have regarding your prescription or insulin should be handled right away. It is on the basis of this relationship between you and your healthcare practitioner that successful treatments and better health results can be provided.

10. Regular Monitoring

Your ability to control your blood sugar levels can be improved by monitoring it. The procedure can be carried out at home using a glucometer, a portable blood glucose meter. With your doctor, you can discuss this possibility.

Consider routinely tracking your levels in a log and recording the results each day. Keeping track of your blood sugar in pairs may also be more beneficial, such as before and after a workout or before and two hours after a meal. You can assess your progress by keeping track and see whether your diet or medicine needs to be changed.

You can also discover how particular meals affect your body's responses. If a meal causes your blood sugar to jump, this can help you determine whether you should make little alterations to it rather than forgoing your favorite foods entirely. Changing a starchy side dish for a vegetable that isn't starchy or limiting the amount to a handful are a few modifications.

11. Uphold a Healthy Weight

Maintaining a healthy weight lowers your chance of developing diabetes and supports good blood sugar levels. According to research, losing 5% of your body weight can even improve blood sugar control and lessen the need for diabetes medication. For instance, if a person who weighs 200 pounds (91 kg) sheds just 10 to 14 pounds (4.5 to 6 kg), their blood sugar levels may significantly improve.

Furthermore, your glycated hemoglobin (HbA1c) values may improve if you lose more than 5% of your starting weight. These serve as a barometer for your blood sugar throughout the last three months.

12. Consume Wholesome Snacks More Often

You may be able to avoid having high or low blood sugar levels by eating small meals and snacks frequently throughout the day, as this will help lower your risk of type 2 diabetes. A number of studies indicate that eating smaller, more frequent meals throughout the day may enhance insulin sensitivity and reduce blood sugar levels.

Additionally, eating more frequent, smaller meals and nutritious snacks throughout the day may result in lower glycated hemoglobin (HbA1c) values, a marker of blood sugar improvements over the past three months.

13. Consume Meals High in Probiotics

Beneficial bacteria known as probiotics have a host of health advantages, including better blood sugar management. According to research, type 2 diabetics who consume probiotics may have a reduction in their HbA1c, insulin resistance, and fasting blood sugar levels. Intriguingly, research has shown that those who take different species of probiotics and do so for at least eight weeks experience greater reductions in blood sugar levels.

Some probiotic-rich foods are as follows:
- tempeh
- sauerkraut
- kefir
- kimchi
- yogurt, as long as the label states that it contains live active cultures
- Miso

14. Consult a Healthcare Provider

Consulting a healthcare professional is crucial if you have diabetes or believe you may have a blood sugar problem. A healthcare specialist can provide individualized guidance based on your particular circumstances, carry out required diagnostic tests, and suggest the best course of action. This could involve making lifestyle adjustments, taking medication, starting insulin therapy, or using a combination of methods to help you effectively manage your illness and advance your wellbeing. You will get the finest care and support for your particular requirements if you keep in regular contact with your healthcare practitioner.

Finally, managing blood sugar levels is a highly individualized journey. Collaborating closely with a healthcare professional is crucial to develop a plan tailored to your unique needs. Your healthcare provider can help you understand your condition, set achievable goals, and recommend lifestyle changes, medication, or insulin therapy as necessary. Regular check-ins and open communication with your healthcare team will ensure that your plan remains effective and adaptable to your evolving health needs. Remember, you're not alone on this journey, and your healthcare provider is there to provide guidance and support every step of the way.

Chapter 5

Creating a Diabetes-Friendly Diet

A healthy lifestyle for someone with diabetes should include both nutrition and exercise. Along with other advantages, maintaining a balanced diet and exercising regularly can assist you in preserving your goal range of blood glucose, often known as blood sugar. You must strike a balance between what you eat and drink, physical exercise, and diabetes medications, if you take them, in order to control your blood sugar. Maintaining your blood glucose level in the range that your medical team advises depends on your choice of food, how much you consume, and when you eat.

Making meals with a mindful balance of nutrients and designing a diet that is diabetes-friendly is similar to becoming the architect of your health. Imagine creating a customized menu: you choose nourishing carbohydrates like whole grains and vegetables while watching portion sizes; you invite lean proteins and the right kinds of fats to the table for stability and satisfaction; you incorporate the superpower of fiber from fruits and vegetables to help regulate blood sugar; and you enjoy the art of portion control while staying hydrated. With the help of this culinary adventure, you'll be able to control your blood sugar levels, turning regular meals into a tasty and proactive way to take care of your health.

Creating a diabetes-friendly diet involves managing carbohydrate intake, choosing whole foods, and monitoring blood sugar levels.

Focus on:

1. Carbohydrates

Control portion sizes and opt for complex carbs like

- *Whole grains*

Includes wheat, rice, oats, cornmeal, barley, and quinoa.
Examples: bread, pasta, cereal, and tortillas.

- *Vegetables*

These include both starchy and non-starchy.
  - Starchy:
Includes potatoes, corn, and green peas
  - Non-starchy:
Includes broccoli, carrots, greens, peppers, and tomatoes

- *Legumes*

Include legumes such as beans, lentils, and chickpeas for fiber and protein.

Note: Half a cup of beans has roughly 115 calories, 20 grams of carbohydrate, 7-9 grams of fiber, 8 grams of protein, and 1 gram of fat per serving. Additionally, the glycemic index of legumes is low, typically falling in the range 10 to 40.

- *Fruits*

Opt for low-sugar fruits like

- oranges, melon,
- pears, berries, apples,
- bananas, and grapes.

2. Protein

Proteins are essential macromolecules composed of amino acids, and they play a crucial role in various biological processes. They are the building blocks of cells, tissues, enzymes, and many other molecules in the body. Protein can be a beneficial part of a diabetic person's diet. Protein-rich diets can help stabilize blood sugar levels and prevent sharp increases by slowing down the absorption of carbohydrates during meals.

They include:

- Lean meat:
    - Lean meats include skinless chicken, skinless turkey, and red meat with the fat removed, like pork chops.
- Fish, eggs, nuts and peanuts
- Dried beans and certain peas, such as chickpeas and split peas
- Meat substitutes, such as tofu
- Dairy (nonfat or low fat):

- Milk or lactose-free milk if you have lactose intolerance
- Yogurt
- Cheese

3. Heart-healthy fats

Heart-healthy fats are crucial for diabetics as they can help control blood sugar levels and lower the risk of cardiovascular problems, which are more common in those with diabetes.

Here are some heart-healthy fats that diabetics can incorporate into their diets:

- Nuts and seeds (almonds, peanuts, cashew, walnuts, flaxseeds, and chia seeds are good sources of healthy fats, fiber, and various vitamins and minerals).
- Fish such as salmon, tuna, trout, and mackerel.
- Avocado
- Canola and olive oil (as they remain liquid at room temperature).
- Coconut Oil: While it's controversial, some people with diabetes find that using coconut oil in moderation can have positive effects on blood sugar.

Note: Instead of using stick margarine, butter, cream, lard, or shortening while cooking, use oils.

4. Stay Hydrated

Drink plenty of water, as dehydration can affect blood sugar levels. Staying hydrated is crucial for individuals with diabetes. Adequate water intake helps regulate blood sugar levels and prevents complications related to dehydration. Water is the best choice for hydration, as it contains no calories or sugars. Monitoring blood sugar regularly, especially when dehydrated, is important.

Aim to drink around 8-10 glasses (about 2-2.5 liters) of water per day, adjusting based on factors like age, activity level, and climate. Be cautious of sugary drinks, and prioritize water during exercise to support blood sugar control and performance. Consulting a healthcare professional can provide personalized hydration recommendations to ensure optimal well-being.

5. Portion Control

A key component of controlling diabetes is portion control. It's critical to pay close attention to the sizes of the food portions you eat in order to successfully control blood sugar levels. Tools that can help you accomplish this aim include measuring cups and cutlery. A portion of protein should roughly be the size of your hand when it comes to lean meats or seafood. Fruit servings are normally similar to a small slice or half a cup, however carbohydrates like grains should be measured in cups. Your dish should consist primarily of non-starchy vegetables. While fats should be used in moderation, a tablespoon of oil or a small handful of nuts is usually a suitable serving size.

6. Glycemic Index Awareness

Glycemic Index (GI) awareness is important for understanding how different foods can affect blood sugar levels. The GI is a numerical scale that ranks carbohydrates in foods based on how quickly they raise blood glucose levels compared to pure glucose. Low-GI foods have a slower impact on blood sugar, while high-GI foods cause a rapid spike.

Being aware of the GI of foods can help individuals with diabetes or those trying to manage their blood sugar levels make informed dietary choices. Low-GI foods like whole grains, fruits, and vegetables are generally better for stabilizing blood sugar, while high-GI foods like sugary snacks and white bread can lead to fluctuations. Promoting GI awareness can encourage healthier eating habits and help people make choices that support their overall health and well-being.

7. Regular Meals

Maintaining a regular eating schedule with balanced meals and snacks is essential for managing blood sugar levels, particularly for individuals with diabetes. Consistency in meal timing helps prevent extreme spikes and drops in blood sugar, promoting better stability throughout the day. Aim for well-rounded meals that include a mix of carbohydrates, proteins, and healthy fats to slow down the absorption of glucose and provide sustained energy. Snacking on nutritious options between meals can also help prevent overeating and keep blood sugar levels steady. Working with a healthcare provider or dietitian to create a personalized meal plan can offer valuable guidance in managing diabetes effectively.

8. Consult a Dietitian

Anyone who wants to effectively manage their disease should consult a qualified dietician who specializes in diabetes. These experts can offer individualized advice on nutrition, meal planning, and lifestyle decisions based on a person's particular requirements and preferences. You can develop a balanced meal plan with the aid of a nutritionist who specializes in diabetes, learn how to make better food choices, and gain insight into how certain foods affect your blood sugar levels. By making it simpler to reach and maintain stable blood sugar levels while enhancing general wellbeing, this cooperative approach can dramatically enhance diabetes management.

9. Monitor Blood Sugar

A crucial part of managing diabetes is keeping a close eye on blood sugar levels as advised by your healthcare practitioner. You can learn a lot about how your body reacts to various foods, activities, and medications by often checking your blood sugar. You may decide what to eat, how often to exercise, and how to take your medications with the help of this information. It's an essential tool for achieving and maintaining stable blood sugar levels, lowering the risk of complications, and making sure your diabetes management strategy continues to work over time. When and how often to check your blood sugar are advised by your healthcare professional, always abide by their advice.

Remember that diabetes management is highly individualized, and what works for one person may not work for another. It's crucial to work closely with your healthcare team to develop a nutrition plan tailored to your specific needs and goals. Balancing these macronutrients depends on your individual needs and health goals. Consulting a registered dietitian can help create a personalized diet plan that meets your specific requirements.

Chapter 6

Foods to Include in Your Diet

Making informed meal choices that maintain blood sugar balance and advance general well-being is essential for managing diabetes. Blood sugar spikes can be avoided by giving low glycemic index foods, like whole grains and non-starchy vegetables, priority. The risk of heart disease can be decreased by incorporating heart-healthy fats from foods like avocados and almonds. Because they suppress hunger and give you long-lasting energy, lean proteins and high-fiber diets aid in weight management. Leafy greens are a nutrient-dense food that provides important vitamins and minerals, helps with digestion, and reduces inflammation.

The best way to ensure a balanced approach that promotes long-term health and diabetes management is to tailor your diet to your particular needs, perhaps with the assistance of healthcare professionals.

Below are the foods to include in your diet plan:

Whole Grains and Lean Proteins

For individuals with diabetes, it's crucial to choose whole grains and lean proteins that have a minimal impact on blood sugar levels. Here's a list:

Whole Grains

1. Quinoa: A complete protein source and rich in fiber.
2. Brown Rice: Higher in fiber and nutrients compared to white rice.
3. Oats: Contain beta-glucans that can help stabilize blood sugar.
4. Barley: Has a low glycemic index and is high in soluble fiber.
5. Bulgur: Quick-cooking and low on the glycemic index.
6. Whole Wheat Pasta: Choose whole grain varieties for more fiber.
7. Farro: A nutrient-dense ancient grain with a good amount of fiber.
8. Millet: A gluten-free grain with a low glycemic index.
9. Whole Grain Bread: Look for 100% whole wheat or whole grain options.

Lean Proteins

1. Skinless Poultry: Chicken and turkey are excellent choices.

2. Fish: Salmon, trout, mackerel, and sardines provide healthy omega-3 fats.

3. Tofu and Tempeh: Plant-based proteins that are low in carbs.

4. Lean Cuts of Meat: If you consume red meat, choose lean cuts like sirloin or tenderloin.

5. Legumes: Beans (e.g., black beans, kidney beans, and lentils) are rich in protein and fiber.

6. Greek Yogurt: High in protein and lower in sugar compared to regular yogurt.

7. Cottage Cheese: Low in carbohydrates and high in protein.

8. Eggs: A great source of protein and essential nutrients.

Remember to control portion sizes and balance your meals with vegetables and healthy fats to help manage blood sugar levels effectively. It's also advisable to work with a healthcare professional or dietitian to create a personalized meal plan that suits your specific needs and preferences.

Healthy Fats and Fiber

Healthy fats and fiber are essential components of a balanced and nutritious diet. Here's why they're important and a list of foods that provide them:

Healthy Fats

- Heart Health: Healthy fats, such as monounsaturated and polyunsaturated fats, can improve heart health by reducing bad cholesterol levels.
- Brain Function: Fats are crucial for brain health and cognitive function.
- Nutrient Absorption: Certain vitamins (like A, D, E, and K) are fat-soluble, meaning they require fat for proper absorption.
- Satiety: Fats help you feel full and satisfied, reducing the urge to overeat.
- Skin and Hair: They contribute to healthy skin and hair.

Sources of Healthy Fats:

1. Avocado: Rich in monounsaturated fats and fiber.
2. Olive Oil: Contains heart-healthy monounsaturated fats.
3. Fatty Fish: Salmon, mackerel, and sardines provide omega-3 fatty acids.
4. Nuts and Seeds: Almonds, walnuts, flaxseeds, and chia seeds are good sources.
5. Nut Butters: Opt for natural peanut or almond butter without added sugars or Trans fats.
6. Coconut: Coconut oil and unsweetened coconut flakes contain healthy fats.

7. Dark Chocolate: In moderation, dark chocolate (70% cocoa or higher) can be a source of healthy fats.

Fiber

- Digestive Health: Fiber aids in regular bowel movements and prevents constipation.
- Blood Sugar Control: It can help stabilize blood sugar levels by slowing the absorption of sugar.
- Weight Management: High-fiber foods promote satiety and can aid in weight control.
- Heart Health: Soluble fiber can lower bad cholesterol levels, reducing the risk of heart disease.
- Gut Health: Fiber feeds beneficial gut bacteria, promoting a healthy microbiome.

Sources of Fiber:

1. Whole Grains: Oats, brown rice, quinoa, and whole wheat.
2. Legumes: Beans, lentils, and chickpeas are rich in fiber and protein.
3. Fruits: Berries, apples, pears, and oranges are high in fiber.
4. Vegetables: Broccoli, Brussels sprouts, carrots, and spinach are fiber-packed.
5. Nuts and Seeds: Almonds, chia seeds, and flaxseeds are good sources.
6. Psyllium Husk: Often used as a fiber supplement.

7. Popcorn: When air-popped without excessive butter or oil.

Incorporating these healthy fats and fiber-rich foods into your diet can contribute to overall well-being and help maintain a balanced and nutritious eating pattern.

Fruits, Vegetables, and Dairy Alternatives

For individuals with diabetes, choosing the right fruits, vegetables, and dairy alternatives is crucial to manage blood sugar levels effectively. Here are some options to consider:

Fruits

1. Berries: Blueberries, strawberries, raspberries, and blackberries are low in sugar and high in antioxidants and fiber.
2. Citrus Fruits: Oranges, grapefruits, and lemons are good choices due to their lower glycemic index.
3. Apples: They provide fiber and are a satisfying, low-glycemic fruit.
4. Pears: Rich in fiber and nutrients, including vitamin K and vitamin C.
5. Kiwi: Low in carbohydrates and high in fiber, vitamin C, and potassium.

6. Cherries: They have a lower glycemic index compared to some other fruits.

Vegetables

1. Leafy Greens: Spinach, kale, and Swiss chard are low in carbohydrates and packed with nutrients.
2. Broccoli: A low-carb vegetable rich in fiber, vitamins, and minerals.
3. Cauliflower: A versatile, low-carb option for mashing, roasting, or making cauliflower rice.
4. Bell Peppers: They add color and nutrients to meals without a significant impact on blood sugar.
5. Zucchini: A low-carb vegetable that can be spiralized into "zoodles" or used in various dishes.

Dairy Alternatives

1. Almond Milk: Unsweetened almond milk is low in carbs and calories.
2. Soy Milk: Provides protein and is a good source of calcium.
3. Coconut Milk: Unsweetened versions are low in carbs.
4. Greek Yogurt (Low-Fat or Non-Fat)**: Higher in protein and lower in sugar compared to regular yogurt.
5. Lactose-Free Dairy: If lactose is an issue, lactose-free cow's milk products are available.

When selecting fruits, be mindful of portion sizes, as they contain natural sugars. Opt for fresh or frozen varieties without added sugars. Additionally, consider your individual response to different foods and monitor your blood sugar levels to determine which options work best for you. Consulting with a healthcare provider or registered dietitian can help create a personalized diabetes management plan tailored to your needs.

Chapter 8

Foods to Avoid or Limit

Avoiding processed foods and foods high in sugar is a good idea for managing diabetes. These troublemakers can cause your blood sugar to soar, giving you the sensation of being on an emotional rollercoaster. Not only are they empty calories, but they also act as yearning magnets, making it difficult to maintain a healthy diet. Not to mention their propensity for gaining weight, which is bad for managing diabetes. Over time, they may increase your risk of developing heart disease and other illnesses. It is best to limit your consumption of certain meals in order to manage your diabetes. Concentrate on full, unprocessed foods like fresh fruits, lean meats, and whole grains since they help you maintain a steady, healthy course and provide better blood sugar management.

Here's why they should be avoided or consumed sparingly:

Sugary Foods

1. Blood Sugar Spikes

Sugary foods and beverages like candy and pastries are frequently referred to as "fast-acting carbohydrates" because they can induce sharp spikes in blood sugar levels, which can be dangerous for those with diabetes. The body may struggle to adequately manufacture or utilise insulin if blood sugar climbs too quickly. In addition to long-term concerns like heart disease, kidney issues, and nerve damage, this can cause immediate symptoms like exhaustion and excessive thirst. Because of this, controlling one's intake of sugary foods is an essential component of diabetes therapy.

2. Empty Calories

Empty calories are obtained from meals and beverages that have little to no nutritional value, meaning that they don't contain any important vitamins, minerals, fiber, or other healthy components. They don't provide your body with the nutrition it needs, which can result in excessive calorie consumption.

Consuming empty calories without any of the nutrients required for healthy blood sugar regulation can be dangerous for someone with diabetes because it can induce blood sugar rises. It is for this reason why emphasizing nutrient-dense foods, such as fruits, vegetables, whole grains, and lean proteins, is so crucial. By giving your body the vital nutrients it requires, these foods not only promote blood sugar control but also general wellness.

3. Cravings

Absolutely, sugary foods have a way of setting off a craving frenzy that can make it really tough to stay on track with a balanced diet. When you indulge in sugary treats, your blood sugar levels skyrocket and then crash, leaving you feeling tired and craving more of that sweet rush. Moreover, these foods activate your brain's pleasure center, making them a tempting choice when emotions run high.

The tricky part is, the more you give in to these cravings, the stronger they become, creating a cycle that's tough to break. To keep your appetite in check and maintain a healthier diet, focusing on foods that provide sustained energy, like whole grains, lean proteins, and healthy fats, can help you avoid those rollercoaster cravings and make better choices for your overall well-being.

Processed Foods

1. High in Added Sugars

When it comes to blood sugar control, hidden sugars in processed foods can be a cunning offender. These hidden added sugars, which can have a disastrous effect on your blood sugar levels, are frequently found in foods that seem harmless, such as cereals, sauces, and snacks. The issue is that they may not always be clear; for example, they may be classified as high fructose corn syrup, maltose, or dextrose.

It can be difficult to keep blood sugar levels constant because these sugars can produce abrupt surges. Because of this, it's critical to become a label detective, looking for unmarked sugars and choosing goods with little to no added sugar. A wise approach to control your blood sugar and promote your health is to select whole, unprocessed foods wherever possible.

2. Excess Sodium

The high sodium content of processed meals might be problematic, especially if you are trying to control your diabetes. These meals' high sodium content can mess with your blood pressure, which could later cause cardiac problems. Because it raises the risk of heart disease and other problems, high blood pressure is a major worry for people with diabetes.

Additionally, a high salt intake might lead to fluid retention, which can make you feel swollen and uneasy. It is advisable to monitor your salt consumption closely because heart health is crucial for people with diabetes. By choosing fresh, whole foods and employing herbs and spices to flavor your home cooking, you can reduce your salt intake and safeguard your heart.

3. Lack of Fiber

Processed foods frequently don't have the necessary fiber for managing diabetes. Being a food that slows down sugar absorption, fiber is important for regulating blood sugar levels in people with diabetes. Additionally, it controls your appetite and aids in maintaining a healthy weight, which is essential for managing your diabetes.

The benefits of fiber for your digestive health, including regularity and the avoidance of constipation, extend beyond blood sugar levels. Think about switching to whole, unprocessed foods high in fiber, such as fresh fruits, vegetables, whole grains, legumes, and nuts, to take control of your diabetes and general health. You'll be giving your body the resources it needs to flourish and efficiently control diabetes if you do this.

4. Unhealthy Fats

In particular for those who are managing diabetes, the prevalence of harmful saturated and hydrogenated fats in processed meals is a real issue. Saturated fats, which are frequently present in certain meals, can elevate LDL (bad) cholesterol levels, raising the risk of heart disease. The much more dangerous hydrogenated fats, often known as Trans fats, are a twofold threat to heart health since they not only raise bad cholesterol but also diminish the good.

These fats act as starting points for the body's inflammatory response, which is a factor in heart disease and other chronic health problems. Avoiding these bad fats is essential for protecting cardiovascular health, especially since people with diabetes already have an increased risk of developing heart disease.

Choose heart-healthy fats instead, which can help you control your diabetes and maintain overall health while preserving the health of your heart. These fats are found in foods like avocados, almonds, and fatty fish.

While it's acceptable to occasionally indulge in sugary or processed treats, it's crucial to do so in moderation. Focusing on complete, unprocessed foods like fruits, vegetables, lean meats, and whole grains is a more efficient strategy for people with diabetes to regulate their blood sugar levels and promote their general health.

Here's a comprehensive list of foods to avoid or limit when managing diabetes:

1. *Sugary Snacks*: Candies, cookies, and sugary cereals.
2. *Sugary Drinks*: Soda, fruit juices, and sweetened beverages.
3. *White Bread and Pasta*: High in refined carbs that spike blood sugar.
4. *Fried Foods*: Deep-fried items like French fries and fried chicken.
5. *Processed Meats*: Bacon, sausage, and processed deli meats, often high in sodium.
6. *Excessive Portions*: Be mindful of portion sizes for all foods.
7. *Sweetened Condiments*: Ketchup, BBQ sauce, and salad dressings with added sugars.
8. *Alcohol*: Drinking can affect blood sugar levels; consume in moderation.
9. *High-Fat Dairy*: Full-fat milk and cheese may be high in saturated fats.
10. *Canned Soups*: Many have high sodium and hidden sugars.
11. *Dried Fruits*: Concentrated sources of sugar; fresh fruits are a better choice.

12. *Candy and Pastries*: Traditional sweets, cakes, and pastries are high in sugar.

13. *Processed Snacks*: Chips, crackers, and packaged snacks often contain unhealthy fats and carbs.

14. *Fast Food*: Burgers, fries, and similar items are typically high in unhealthy fats and carbs.

15. *Saturated and Trans Fats*: Limit foods with high levels of these fats, like some margarines and baked goods.

16. *High-Sugar Breakfast Cereals*: Opt for whole-grain, low-sugar options.

17. *Flavored Yogurts*: Often contain added sugars; choose plain or low-sugar versions.

18. *Instant Noodles*: High in sodium and refined carbs.

19. *High-Sugar Sauces*: Some pasta sauces and Asian sauces can be high in sugar.

20. *Energy Drinks*: Loaded with sugar and caffeine, they can disrupt blood sugar control.

Managing diabetes is all about making smart food choices to keep your blood sugar stable. Prioritizing whole, unprocessed foods and being mindful of sugar and carb content can go a long way in helping you maintain good health.

Conclusion

In the last sections of "Diabetes and Diet: The Road to Blood Sugar Control," we've set out on a quest to comprehend the complex connection between diet and diabetes control. Remember that this book is only the beginning as we come to an end on this educational journey. Knowledge, decisions, and willpower all play a part in the continual journey toward blood sugar control. With the knowledge you've received in these pages, you're prepared to adopt a healthy lifestyle, make wise nutritional choices, and successfully deal with the difficulties associated with diabetes. Your tenacity and dedication to wellbeing are demonstrated by your journey towards better blood sugar management. On this journey to a healthier, more balanced existence, keep learning, keep changing, and keep thriving.

Good luck!

References

https://idf.org/about-diabetes/what-is-diabetes/

https://pubmed.ncbi.nlm.nih.gov/31518657/

https://pubmed.ncbi.nlm.nih.gov/34749892/

https://www.diabetes.co.uk/food/lean-meat.html

https://www.diabetes.org.uk/diabetes-the-basics/types-of-diabetes

https://www.diabetesselfmanagement.com/managing-diabetes/blood-glucose-management/blood-sugar-chart/

https://www.healthline.com/nutrition/14-ways-to-lower-blood-sugar#TOC_TITLE_HDR_4

https://www.medicalnewstoday.com/articles/317458#

https://www.ncbi.nlm.nih.gov/pmc/articles/PMC4608274/

https://www.niddk.nih.gov/health-information/diabetes/overview/diet-eating-physical-activity

https://www.signos.com/blog/spices-that-may-lower-blood-sugar

https://www.vecteezy.com/free-photos/blood-glucose

https://www.who.int/health-topics/diabetes

www.ingramcontent.com/pod-product-compliance
Lightning Source LLC
Chambersburg PA
CBHW060755260726
48660CB00002B/631